ISBN 978-0-9930695-4-3

Published by:

Bardic Media
Unit 601
10 Southgate Road
London
N1 3LY

Simply Parkinson's

**Written and illustrated
by
John Duncan**

John Duncan is a former banker, public relations executive, freelance journalist, broadcaster and commentator and is the author of *Cricket Wonderful Cricket* and *How to Manage your Bank Manager.*

Now 82, he was diagnosed with Parkinson's in 2009 and lives in London & Catalunya with his wife, Helen, who cares for him, while he writes and draws and keeps on keeping on.

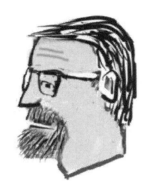

To Kate and Anna who made George
a very proud Grandpop!

Simply Parkinson's

by John Duncan

Contents

Foreword 9

Chapter One....... .*Early signs* 13

Chapter Two....... *Symptoms* 17

Chapter Three .... *Treatments*....................... 25

Chapter Four ...... *Feelings* 29

Chapter Five .... *Help* 35

Afterword.. 39

Thanks.. 43

Foreword

How many people have Parkinson's Disease? How do they get it? What is it like to suffer from it? Is there a cure? And is there anything that can be done to help?

There are no simple answers to these questions for it is a complex complaint which very few people fully understand. It is one of the most significant medical mysteries that creates a life that can be impossible to control. But in other cases, with the right medication, a life can continue to be close to normal.

An estimated seven to ten million people worldwide are living with Parkinson's Disease. These include, or once included: Roger Bannister, Billy Connolly, Salvador Dali, Neil Diamond, Michael J Fox, Billy Graham, Bob Hoskins, Kenneth More, Muhammad Ali, Enoch Powell, Sir Michael Redgrave, Linda Ronstadt and Terry-Thomas.

There are estimated to be 145,000 sufferers in the United Kingdom alone; that is one in every 350 adults. Every hour another person (who is likely to be over 60) is told that they have the disease. And the chances are that they will be male rather than female.

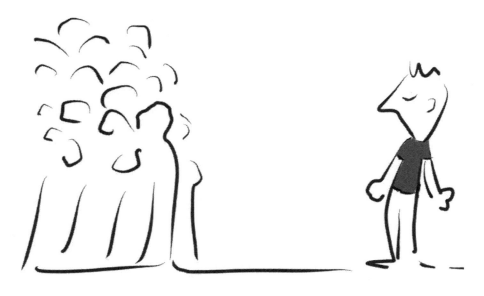

One in 350

But what is Parkinson's? I have tried to explain here, in simple terms, firstly what the disease involves and its impact on so many peoples' lives. And secondly, to make it easier to understand by anyone having contact with a sufferer, particularly for the first time.

Chapter One - Early signs

Parkinson's Disease (or PD as I will refer to it throughout) is not easy to diagnose, particularly for an overworked GP who cannot be expected to differentiate between PD and other conditions which can cause a patient to shake in one way or another. This can mean, of course, that a correct diagnosis may not be made until PD has already been active for some time.

The earliest signs can vary but shaking or tremors in one hand or arm is very common and frequently dropping things and difficulty in walking with normal strides is not unusual. A neurological expert will carry out a series of physical tests which are quite simple but make it possible to evaluate whether or not this is a case of the real thing.

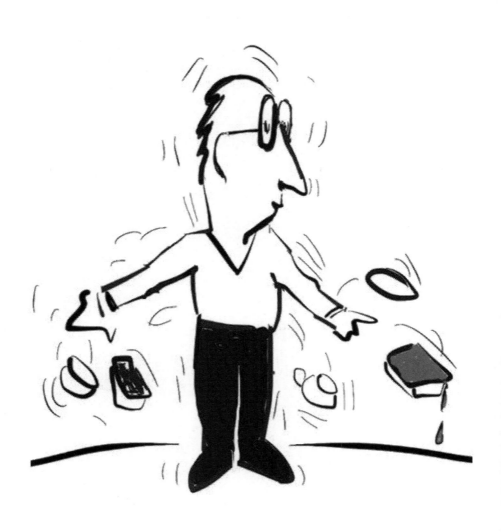

Shaking or tremors

If this is so, then decisions must be made regarding the appropriate treatment for the patient, based on the stage in the development of his or her PD.

But how does someone come to have PD in the first place? Is it contagious? Is it hereditary? There are no easy answers to the reason why one person has the disease and another does not. Lifestyle in the form of drinking heavily or smoking, over-eating or lack of exercise are not thought to be involved as they are in many other cases of ill-health.

There has been no solid evidence of it being passed down from one generation to another even though it is not unknown for a parent, offspring or other relatives to suffer. You cannot catch it like the common cold or influenza.

Which means that there are really no established reasons for becoming afflicted. It has been suggested that pesticides are a cause, but this is just one possible answer.

But what is known is that the problem starts in certain nerve cells in the brain that are meant to produce a chemical called Dopamine but do not do so. Dopamine is vital as a messenger, in effect, telling our body what to do and without it we are not able to control properly a wide range of bodily functions that would normally not be a problem.

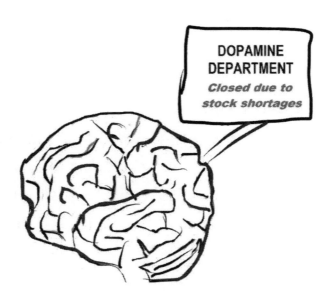

Chapter Two - Symptoms

There are many symptoms and side effects involved in PD. These are a strange mixture of challenges for a sufferer, both physical and mental, which can be evident in one case and not in another. In other words, once someone has PD it is not necessarily going to be the case that they will be burdened with the same symptoms as the next person in the queue. And the impact and frequency of one ingredient can be and often is very different.

In chapter four I talk about feelings, emotions and what it can be like to have PD. However, right here you will find a shopping list of symptoms and more comprehensive coverage of this aspect is available elsewhere. For example, look online for michaeljfox.org, a charity based in the USA which is an excellent source.

In the UK, the two charities in particular with websites well worth a visit can be found at parkinsons.org.uk and cureparkinsons.org.uk. They do tremendous work in funding research and providing information and if you are in the position of being able to make charitable donations they would welcome your support. And if you really want to dig and delve, search for Parkinson's at nice.org.uk.

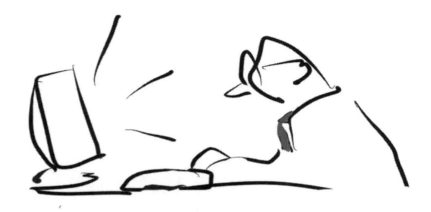

Websites well worth a visit

Then there are search engines, such as Google, that will help you to find an enormous amount of information much of which is practical and helpful, although to be quite honest some of it is totally incomprehensible. Some of the symptoms and medications appear to be written about in a language that is foreign to us all. But then again I'm not a fully qualified neurologist. Not yet at least...

However, I digress. Back to the shopping list. In no particular order (now where have I heard that before?) it's what you simply may not find elsewhere in other chapters. And it is important to understand that while many of these symptoms and conditions are directly as a result of PD, a fair number can be caused by the medication taken to treat or control it.

✳ *Movement*

Probably the best place to start is at the very heart of what this is all about. It covers a number of key areas directly relating to the way the body behaves. These include balance, rigidity, mobility, freezing, shuffling, posture, gait and turning. In effect the body no longer behaves in the way that it used to.

It is almost as though it has a mind of its own over which there is no control. So for some it brings with it the feeling that at any moment you might fall, when it is as though your

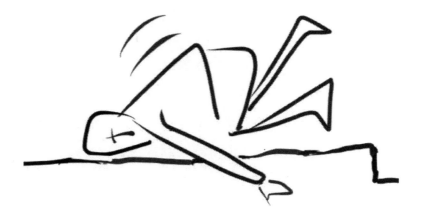

Fear of falling

muscles have turned to stone, when you cannot walk properly, when you cannot turn around and when you cannot stand upright.

✳ **Tremors**

Where it all begins, usually on one side, in fingers, hand or arm. Then spreads.

✳ *Sleeping and Restless Leg Syndrome*

Plenty in store here, not least difficulties
getting in and out of bed. Once in there, like a
beached whale, it is difficult to roll or turn over.
Then while you're lying there, minding your
own business, you start perspiring as though
in a sauna. Then, for no apparent reason, your
leg or legs start to twitch and jerk
unpredictably and uncontrollably. Welcome to
Restless Leg Syndrome. And, despite
medication, goodbye sleep.

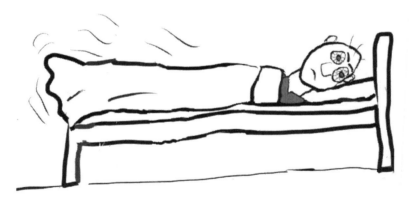

And goodbye sleep

✳ *Mind*

Anxiety – can be quite common and vary in intensity. Even the smallest of concerns can create a disproportionate level of anxiety.

Hallucinations - not unusual to see, hear or feel things that don't actually exist.

Delusions - worrying or thinking about things that are not real.

Compulsive behaviour - can include shopping, hoarding, eating, gambling. In some cases, can become a very difficult problem to deal with.

✳ *Physical*

Skin conditions - the surface of all parts of the body can become dry, flaky, oily or develop a rash.

Bowels and bladder - various difficulties can arise, often unpredictably, often urgently. Constipation is quite common and diarrhoea is not unusual.

Sexual dysfunction - what used to be enormous fun, sometimes now just can't be done.

Voice - muscles involved in speech can be affected so that it becomes quieter.

Face - facial expressions can disappear. Sufferers can look miserable when they are not.

Vision - eyes can become tired and watery, vision blurred as well as other sight related problems.

Handwriting - once you were able to write clearly, perhaps even stylishly. Now all that you can produce is a messy mass of muddled indecipherable meanderings.

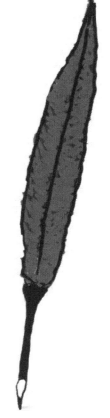

No longer write clearly

Chapter Three -Treatments

As things stand currently and have done ever since PD was first identified, there is no known cure. But research is intense and there is progress with new solutions and the adaptation of other medication that has originally been effective in the treatment of unrelated illnesses.

In the meantime, it is a matter of controlling the condition in the best way possible and as each individual with PD is different, so will the treatment need to be. This may be a combination of medication with additional benefits gained from alternative therapies and exercise. The aim is to get the balance right so as to make life as bearable as possible for the sufferer and to adjust levels of pills and potions as the impact of PD increases. There are a number of types of medication that can help either alone or together by replacing the elusive missing Dopamine or making it more effective in treating, in particular, the physical side of things. Leaving the more confusing and remote medical terms to one side, typical brand names for these drugs are Sinemet and Ropinirole. There is also a number of drugs that help to control other symptoms such as depression, anxiety, constipation and so forth. Unfortunately, some of the medication can and does cause side effects, including several of those listed in the previous chapter.

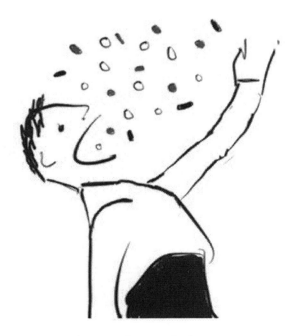

A number of drugs

Surgical therapies are also available, particularly Deep Brain Stimulation, which involves electrical pulses delivered to the brain via a device similar to a pacemaker. It is sometimes used where a patient is responding to medication but has significant 'off' periods.

There is also a wide range of non-medical therapies that can be of assistance. This includes physiotherapy to help with balance and gait and speech therapy to help with speaking or swallowing problems. Acupuncture and massage may provide pain relief and for many people, increasing exercise can be hugely beneficial.

Fun ways to increase exercise depending on your tastes are dancing, Pilates, Shiatsu and many more.

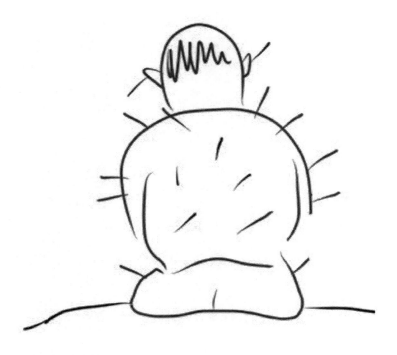

Acupuncture may provide pain relief

Chapter Four - Feelings

So what is it like to have PD? Not an easy question to answer. This is my personal view because clearly individuals have differing feelings based on their own experiences. Nevertheless I am aware of the thoughts of many fellow sufferers so as to ensure that what you will find here is not just the condition of a one trick pony.

So far, this has been an attempt to explain PD in simple rather than medical or neurological terms but the challenge for the sufferer is, all else apart, an emotional one. Perhaps like the ingredients in a cake or the components of a car, they, like the symptoms I have described, are facts. But driving a car or eating cake is probably not a particularly emotional experience. Living with PD undoubtedly is.

No matter how strong minded, positive and optimistic an individual tries to be, it is almost impossible to avoid feeling down for much of the time.

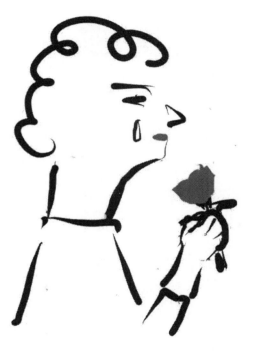

No longer smell a rose

You are living in a world where you cannot control your mind or body in a normal way. What has always come naturally no longer does. You cannot walk properly (I call this my Womble walk!), you drop things, can't do up your shoelaces and can no longer smell a rose. Your mood, your energy, your levels of pain can change without warning.

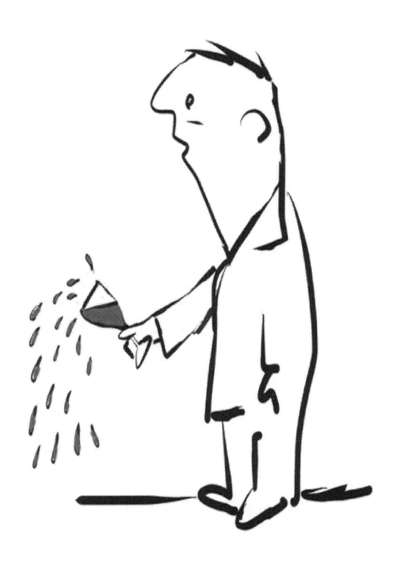

Spill your drink

It is difficult at social events to circulate, at dinner not to distribute your food in all directions, hard to get up from a chair unaided, easy to spill your drink. And you can appear to be drunk or to have gone to the toilet forever. It is quite possible to give the impression that you are not normal.

And it is perhaps as a result of all this it can feel easier and preferable to be on your own and to not have to communicate. Consequently, you can be rude to those who help and love you.

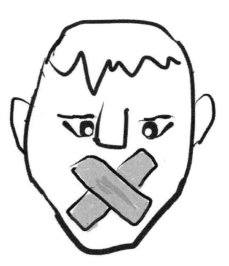

Not communicating

So people do not know how to treat you, what to say, when to help you and when to leave you alone. You aim to be honest about how you are feeling when asked but try not to dwell on it. Those closest to you want to know how you really are; acquaintances may prefer not to!

It is hard work and emotionally exhausting to put on a brave face all the time; as though you are an actor who is permanently performing. There is always the need to find space, physically and emotionally, or to let off steam, that can be anything from a good cry to a few well chosen words unsuitable for those of a sensitive nature!

Nothing is going to change all this but there is a chance that if people have a better understanding of PD and the causes, symptoms and emotions involved, then this may help.

Chapter Five - Help

As PD progresses it is likely that there will be the need for help to be available at some stage. But the rate of development of the disease varies considerably and many sufferers need little or no care or assistance and continue to lead a normal life or something close to it. Many continue working for years after first being diagnosed.

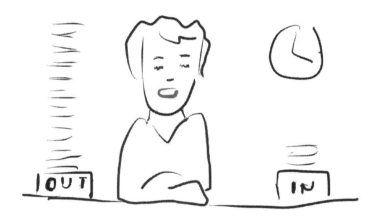

Continue working for many years

Help and information is available from many sources, face-to-face at one end of the scale and online at the other. The GP is, of course, a good starting point and in my experience, the NHS has been enormously supportive. The Neurology specialists, the Parkinson's nurses and others involved are impressive and sensitive to sufferers' needs.

In the UK, there is also the charity that I mentioned earlier, Parkinson's UK, offering useful information, advice and help.

In fact, once personal help is needed, this will often be provided by a member of the family, frequently the spouse. If this assistance is not available, it is worth contacting the local authority who can sometimes help or there are inevitably a number of organisations offering caring services but they do come at a price.

Caring is demanding and variable, something that is difficult to set out in a job description. It calls for delicate judgment on when to help and when to hold back.

The carer has to avoid helping too much or too little by finding the difficult middle position when letting the PD sufferer do it for themselves. Even though it would be a lot quicker to help them getting out of bed, putting on shoes or making a cup of tea, a sense of achievement for them is sometimes more important.

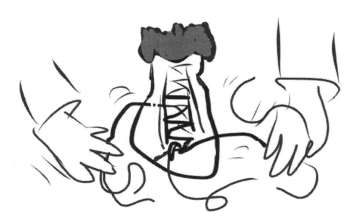

Putting on shoes

This can result in frustration which can lead to the sufferer being unpleasant and unkind. It is a major challenge for the carer not to take it personally and, in particular:

- To know there will be days when the person with PD is really miserable, and there is nothing you can do.
- Learning to cope with the rollercoaster that is PD; never knowing what to expect from hour to hour and day to day.
- Realising that despite your best care, you cannot cure Parkinson's.

Which means that the carer must be able to find both emotional support when they are providing care and respite, a sensible break away from caring, to relax and recharge their batteries.

Afterword

I have been fortunate in many ways particularly because PD has not affected my ability to communicate and to create. Physically I'm not a bundle of laughs and mobility is a particular challenge.

It's easy to get depressed; those black times that seem to creep up on you when you're not looking. Laughter helps combat this and music too. I so enjoy an episode of Frasier, revel in the humour of fellow-sufferer and comedian, Billy Connolly and crease up to Lee Mack. Then swing to Glenn Miller, jazz it up with Louis Armstrong or join in the chorus of Don't Give Up with Peter Gabriel. I exercise when possible, read a book, watch endless sport on TV, produce the most awful noise from a borrowed trombone, eat, drink and be merry.

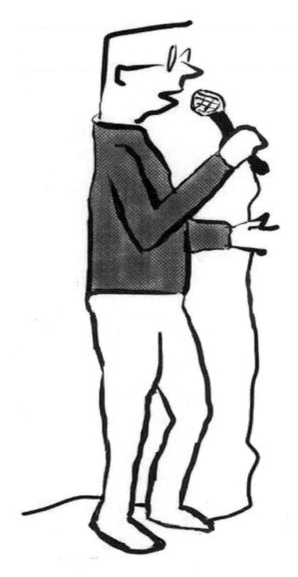

Jazz it up with Louis

And I must say that I find it very helpful to have a creative project, such as this publication, on the go. Being motivated in this way, working towards a goal, seems to really help me.

I am blessed above all with a wonderful wife, marvellous family and friends and the specialists and therapists and many other people who help me in so many ways to deal with PD.

And although I am confident that one day there will be a cure I know, that for me, it is not going to go away. It is progressively degenerative. That means that it is going to get steadily worse. You don't die from PD – you die with it.

But I will keep on keeping on. Enjoying the memories and enjoying the now. And I will not be f****d about by some mysterious irritating triviality. Because of one thing I am absolutely sure...

There are still very many bigger fish yet to be fried before I've had my chips!

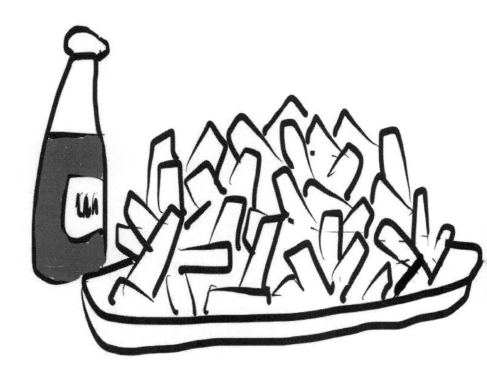

Before I've had my chips

Thanks to my wife, Helen, whose research, contributions, encouragement, understanding, care and love has helped me to complete this publication. To my son, Ged, whose publishing skills saved me from the seriously hard bits. To those kind people who read my drafts and provided guidance and invaluable suggestions.

And thank you to these and many more people who have shown all the care, kindness, assistance and support which enables me to keep on keeping on.

Printed in Great Britain
by Amazon